THE NEW EMT SURVIVAL GUIDE

The Unwritten Manual for a Career in EMS

James Mazza

2026

Published 2026

Printed in the United States of America

Foreword

There is no shortage of material designed to prepare you for a career in Emergency Medical Services.

Textbooks. Training manuals. Certification courses. Online modules with multiple choice questions and progress bars. All of it has its place and none of it will fully prepare you for what this career actually feels like from the inside.

That is why this book exists.

What you are holding is not a textbook. It will not teach you how to assess a patient, manage an airway, or treat a patient in shock. There are plenty of resources for that and you will spend a significant portion of your training working through them. What those resources will not tell you is what it is like to stand next to a dying person on your second shift. What it does to your back after fifteen years of lifting. What it costs the people who love you. What it gives you that nothing else can.

I wrote this because nobody handed it to me when I started and I spent years learning things the hard way.

If you are considering this profession, read this before you decide. Not to be frightened away from it but to walk in with your eyes open.

If you are already on your way, read this as a companion to your training. The clinical skills matter enormously. So does everything in these pages.

And if you have never ridden in the back of an ambulance but have wondered what people experience on the other side of that door, this book is for you too. EMS providers are not heroes in the way the television version suggests. They are human beings doing an extraordinarily difficult job in conditions that most people would not tolerate, for compensation that does not reflect the work, out of a sense of purpose that is genuinely hard to explain to anyone who has not felt it.

I should be honest that I am only one voice in this. Not everyone in this profession feels the way I do about it. Some are here for a paycheck and nothing more, and some would tell you a very different story than the one in these pages. What I can offer you is my truth after close to twenty years, not the truth for everyone who has ever worn the patch.

I have been doing this for close to twenty years. I am the Chief of EMS at Montclair Ambulance Unit, a two-time award-winning EMS administrator, and a member of NJ Task Force 1 Urban Search and Rescue and the New Jersey

EMS Task Force, having deployed to disasters across the country. I have spent nearly two decades working at the local, county, and state level to try to make this profession better. I still cannot fully explain why I keep coming back to it. But I can tell you the truth about it.

That is what I have tried to do here.

The chapters ahead are not always comfortable to read. They were not always comfortable to write. But if you are going to do this work, or if you are trying to understand the people who do, you deserve the truth more than you deserve comfort.

Turn the page.

Chapter 1: Your First Call Will Mess With You

I still have the photos my mom took before my first shift.

I was standing on the front steps of our house, holding an oversized hand-me-down coat with reflective strips that made me look like I had just walked off the set of the TV show *Emergency*. Not wearing it. Holding it. Because it did not fit and I did not care, and I was already annoyed that she was making me stop and pose when I wanted to get moving. I have always hated having my picture taken. I have always preferred to live in the moment rather than document it.

My dad was not there for those photos. He was at his second job, the one he worked to keep the family afloat. He worked the way I would come to work, constantly, because that was what was required. I got that from him. Standing on those steps in my new uniform, I didn't yet understand the price you pay for that. I would spend years learning that lesson.

I did not even have a CPR card when I showed up for that first shift. I was a brand-new volunteer with a spotless uniform, someone else's coat, and a head full of ideas about this job that had been built almost entirely by television. *Rescue 911* was the show that stuck with me most. William

Shatner narrating dramatic rescues, lives hanging in the balance, providers doing extraordinary things in extraordinary moments. That was the template I had constructed. That was what I thought I was walking into.

What I walked into was a rig check.

If you do not know what a rig check is yet, you will learn soon enough, and your feelings about it will evolve over your career in ways you cannot predict right now. A rig check is the systematic inspection of every piece of equipment on the ambulance before your shift begins. Every supply, every device, every medication, every piece of gear accounted for and verified. It is one of the most tedious things you will ever have to do. It is also one of the most important. The call where something is missing is the call that will teach you this lesson permanently, if you have not already learned it. But standing there on my first shift, going through that checklist item by item, this was not what I had signed up for. Where was the action? Where was the drama? Where was William Shatner?

We did not even finish the rig check before the first call came in.

An elderly male who needed help getting up. That was it. That was my first EMS experience. A man, partially undressed, in the kind of physical and personal diminishment that age brings to all of us eventually, who needed help getting off the floor. It wound up being a transport. We helped him, we got him to where he needed to go, and we came back.

I remember the smell more than anything else. I remember the way the apartment looked. I remember thinking that this person had lived an entire life, had probably done remarkable things, had people who loved him, and was now here. Aging is ugly. It is unglamorous and uncomfortable and it strips people of the version of themselves they spent a lifetime building. It comes for all of us. That first call put a face on that reality in a way nothing had before.

I remember standing there thinking nobody had warned me it would look like this.

I was going to be a hero. I was going to hang upside down cutting people out of cars. I was going to deliver a baby on the side of the road. I was going to do the things William Shatner narrated with that voice over dramatic music. Instead I had helped an old man off the floor of his apartment on a Monday night. The gap between what I had imagined and what I had just experienced was significant.

And here's the thing:

That first call was not the exception. It was the preview. The car extractions and the deliveries and the cardiac arrests you bring back do happen. Some of them will happen to you. But they will not be your Monday nights. Your Monday nights will look a lot more like that first call than anything you have seen on television.

Lift assists. Intoxicated patients. Elderly people who are lonely or cold or out of food and do not have anyone else to call. That is the job. Not every shift, but most of them.

We sell this profession on its most dramatic moments because the dramatic moments are what get people in the door. I understand that. But it does a disservice to every new provider who walks in expecting *Rescue 911* and finds themselves doing a rig check at eleven o'clock on a Monday. The expectation gap is where burnout begins. It starts before you even take your first call.

So here is what I am asking you to do before you go any further in this book or any further in this career: Leave the TV version at the door. Not because the heroic moments do not exist—they do and they will find you— but because they are not the whole story and they are not even most of the story.

If you can walk in with clear eyes and honest expectations, your first call will still mess with you. It messed with me and I have been doing this for close to twenty years. But it will not break you. And that is the difference between a first call and a last call.

Chapter 2: You Are Going to Screw Up

Let me get this out of the way early.

You will make mistakes in this career. Not *might*. *Will*. Every day an estimated 700 to 1000 people in the United States die from medical errors. This profession demands perfection because lives depend on it. That standard is real and you should hold yourself to it every single shift. And yet perfection is not something that exists in emergency medicine or anywhere else humans are involved. The demand for it and the inevitability of falling short of it are both true at the same time. If you cannot make peace with that reality, this career will eat you alive.

Here is the part nobody says out loud: Most of your mistakes will not hurt anyone. You will be lucky far more often than you are good, especially early in your career. That is exactly what makes the mistakes dangerous. Every time you get away with one, it teaches you the stakes are not real. They are. The distance between the mistake that costs nothing and the mistake that costs everything is often just luck and timing. What matters is what you do with the mistake after it happens, while the cost is still nothing. A rig check mistake is how most providers first learn this lesson, and almost every experienced EMT has a version of it.

We talk about rig checks in Chapter 1 because they are the foundation of preparedness. You check the truck before every shift so you'll know what you have when you need it. It sounds simple. It is not foolproof. About fifteen years into my career, well past the point where I thought I had this particular lesson mastered, I learned that again.

We had done our rig check. Everything was accounted for. Then we pulled the jump kit off the stretcher to show a piece of equipment to a new employee. We got a call. We went. I grabbed the stairchair, made patient contact, and it was immediately clear this was going to be an RMA, a refusal of medical assistance. The patient had been nervous, wanted some reassurance, wanted someone to check their blood pressure. Nothing serious. I asked my partner for a BP cuff. He walked in holding an oxygen bottle and a BVM and just shook his head.

We had left the jump kit back at the building.

We still had everything we needed to manage the call. It just was not organized and ready to go the way it should have been. We made it work. No harm to the patient that time, and that is the part I want you to sit with. Fifteen years in and there I was, standing in someone's living room having made the exact mistake I had watched rookies make at the beginning of my career. It does not matter how long you have been doing this. The moment you stop treating the rig check like it matters is the moment it will bite you.

Now let me tell you about a bigger mistake.

I was working with a new agency in an area I had never worked before. I had a critically sick patient and was transporting to the hospital. My partner told me where to meet paramedics en route, line of sight on the way in. I followed the GPS, one of those old dashboard mounted ones, and thought I was going the right direction. I was a block over from where I should have been. We never connected with those paramedics. The patient's status did not change, so no actual harm was done. But that was luck, not skill. If that patient had crashed in the block between where I was and where I should have been, this would be a very different story.

When we got to the hospital the paramedics were waiting. They pulled me aside in the ER and tore into me. In front of everyone. Loud and pointed and not remotely constructive. Was I wrong? Yes. Did I know it before they opened their mouths? Also yes. Was the correction warranted? Absolutely. Was that the right way to deliver it? Not even close.

I walked out of that ER thinking two things simultaneously. First, I was never going to let that happen again and I was going to learn every road in that area until I knew it cold. Second—and I will be honest with you, because this book is not about pretending EMS providers are saints —I was thinking some version of what anyone thinks when they get dressed down in front of a room full of people. I was angry. That anger sat with me for a while.

Eventually I let it go. I crossed paths with that paramedic again over the years and we moved past it the way you move past most things in this profession. You carry it, you process it, and at some point you put it down. But it took time and it was a lesson in more than just geography.

What I learned from that call was not just to know my routes. I learned that how we correct the people around us when they make mistakes is just as important as the correction itself. That paramedic was right about the mistake and wrong about the method. Both of those things can be true at the same time. And when it is your turn to be the one doing the correcting (and it will be your turn someday), remember what it felt like to be on the other end of it done badly.

Nobody in this profession will ever make zero mistakes. Not the paramedic who yelled at me in that ER. Not the supervisors who trained you. Not the providers you will eventually look up to. The goal is not to be perfect. The goal is to build a practice that makes the mistakes as small and as rare as possible, to be honest when they happen, and to learn something from every single one of them without letting the weight of them break you. Not avoiding every mistake. Making sure that when the unavoidable ones come, your habits keep them small, so the day luck is not on your side, your practice is.

Chapter 3: Patients Aren't the Hard Part

Your training will prepare you to manage a patient. The textbooks will teach you what interventions to provide when someone presents with a specific condition. Experience will teach you the difference between a patient who is sick and a patient who is not sick. What nobody prepares you for is everything happening around the patient while you are trying to do all of that.

The external factors are harder than the patient. I need you to understand that before your first shift.

Let me tell you about a call in a mall food court.

A child had seized. His mother had administered his prescribed rectal anti-seizure medication before we arrived, which meant his pants were down when my crew got to him. My crew was attending to him when I looked up from the scene and along the second-floor railing, all the way around the food court, there were people filming. Phones out, pointed down at a child who was partially undressed and in the middle of a medical emergency.

I looked up and said it loudly enough for all of them to hear. How would you like it if that was your kid down here and someone was filming your child?

I got some nasty looks. One person talked back. Mall security arrived quickly and cleared the area.

That is what crowd management actually looks like in practice. It is not a clinical skill. It is a human one. You are reading a scene full of people, figuring out what they need to hear, and saying it in a way that moves them. Sometimes it works cleanly. Sometimes it does not. But the alternative is doing nothing and letting the chaos close in around your patient.

My general rule on scene is to control what I can control. As a street provider that means getting the patient into the ambulance as soon as medically practical. Close the doors and you have created your own environment. The noise stays outside. The crowd stays outside. The ambulance becomes the one place on that scene where you are in charge of what happens. That is not always possible and it is not always the right move, but use it when it is available to you.

When you cannot close the doors, you talk. Most of this job is talking to people. You learn to take histories from patients who want to tell you about a hip replacement from twenty years ago when they called you for chest pain. That same skill works on families, on bystanders, on anyone standing between you and the ability to do your job. Meet them where they are emotionally. Do not get tunnel vision. And once you have them calm, figure out how to make them useful.

That last part is important. A family that is no longer panicking is a resource. They know the patient's history, their medications, what led up to the call. A calm bystander can help you manage a crowd. The people around your scene are not always obstacles. Sometimes they are assets you have not activated yet.

Now let me talk about the tension that plays out on almost every call where a patient has family present.

Families want their loved ones to go to the hospital. Not always because the patient needs to go. Sometimes because the person caring for them is exhausted and has been doing it alone for a long time. Sometimes because they are scared and the hospital feels like the safest answer even when it is not. And sometimes the patient does not want to go at all. Bridging that gap is one of the most genuinely difficult things you will do in this career and there is no clean formula for it.

I have used families to help convince patients who genuinely needed the ER to go when they were resistant. I have also had to gently remind families that what they want for their loved one and what their loved one actually needs are not always the same thing. Both of those conversations are hard. Both require you to be present and honest and careful with people who are frightened.

During COVID I responded to a call for an Alzheimer's patient. The family needed a break. Before the pandemic, that was manageable. A transport to the hospital, some respite time, a reset. But during COVID I had to look that family in the eye and tell them plainly that if their loved one went to the hospital there was no guarantee they would ever be able to speak to them again or see them again. COVID had changed everything about what a hospital visit meant for a vulnerable patient.

They still wanted the transport.

I do not know the outcome of that call. I never found out. That is true of most 911 calls. You arrive, you do your job, you leave, and the rest of the story belongs to someone else. What I want you to take from that story here is that the patient autonomy conversation is never simple. Not when someone is in crisis, not when their family is in the room, and not when the world outside has changed the stakes of the decision being made.

You cannot control what families feel. You can control how you show up in those moments.

Everything I just described, reading a scene, controlling what you can control, turning chaos into order, is a muscle you build on ordinary calls so it is there on the worst one. Crowd management is controlling chaos on a routine call. What comes next is controlling chaos when the scene itself is the emergency.

The calls that reveal who you really are as a provider are not the quiet ones. They are the mass casualty incidents, the large-scale events, the scenes where multiple things are happening simultaneously and someone has to hold the whole picture together. You cannot predict when one of those calls is coming. What you can do is prepare for it every single day.

A two-car collision with multiple patients? Call for EMS Branch. Utilize triage tags if the situation warrants them. Working a planned event like a street fair with tens of thousands of people? Draw up an Event Action Plan. Fill out your ICS forms. Practice operating under a unified command structure. These are not bureaucratic exercises. They are the habits that determine how you perform when things go sideways and there is no time to think.

If your agency does not do these things, ask why. Is it a resource issue? A training gap? Is it simply that nobody has pushed for it yet? Work to change that if you can. The mindset is simple even when the execution is not. Practice how you play. Every call is a chance to build the habits that will hold when the big one comes.

Because it will come. And when it does, you will either be ready or you will not. The difference is built on every ordinary call you took seriously before it arrived.

Chapter 4: The Stuff That Sticks With You

At some point in your career, probably at a party or a family dinner, someone is going to ask you what the worst thing you have ever seen is. They will lean in when they ask it. They think they want to know.

Early in my career I answered that question honestly. I was the story person in my college friend group. Every week someone wanted new material and I delivered. I thought I was processing by talking about it. What I was actually doing was reopening the same wounds over and over again in front of people who wanted to be entertained by them. The things I did not want to think about stayed in my mind longer than they should have because I kept pulling them back out and handing them to people who had no idea what they were actually holding.

Now when someone asks me that question I laugh and say, "You do not really want to know! Those images are not ones you want in your head. Let me tell you about the time we helped save someone's life instead."

That shift took years to make. I want you to make it faster than I did.

Here is the truth about the stuff that sticks with you. It is not always what you expect. You will prepare yourself for the big calls, the dramatic ones, the ones that announce themselves as significant from the moment you get the dispatch. What you cannot prepare for is which specific detail lodges in your brain and refuses to leave. It is rarely the one you would expect. I worked a call involving a pedestrian and a bus. What a bus does to a human body is something I will not describe here in detail because there is no reason to put it in your head before you have to carry it yourself. What I will tell you is that we were on scene for more than four hours. The investigation had to run its course. The bus had to be lifted by our team before the coroner could access the body. And so we stood around. We talked with other members of the organization, with police, with fire. We stood in the cold wishing we were anywhere else, home with a book or a cigar or anything that was not this. Time moves strangely at a scene like that. It stretches.

And then the coroner crawled out from under the bus. He stood up, *put his gloved hand on his chin,* a glove that was not clean by any definition of that word, and shook his head. "I don't know how we are going to get him out," he said.

It was one of the most awkward, disgusting, and genuinely absurd moments I have witnessed in this career. I did not know whether to be horrified or to laugh. I felt both simultaneously. If you have read this far you already know that is not an unusual place to find yourself in EMS.

That street exists in the town where I live. I avoided it for months after that call. Not consciously at first. My route just kept not going that way until I noticed I was doing it. The stuff that sticks with you is geographic sometimes. It lives in specific intersections, specific parking lots, specific hallways in specific buildings. You will develop your own map of places you start to avoid. That is normal. It fades eventually, mostly, though some of it never leaves entirely.

Then there are the things that change without you noticing until they already have.

When I started in this profession I had a strong tolerance for the physical realities of emergency medicine. Blood, vomit, feces, the smells that come with bodies and illness and neglect. None of it bothered me. I was fine walking into a nursing home, that specific combination of smells that anyone who has worked in long term care will recognize immediately, the illness and the age and sometimes the death all layered together. I could compartmentalize all of it without much effort.

Twenty years in, that has changed. Sometimes the smell of feces or the sight of vomit makes me want to vomit myself. I do not know exactly why. Too much exposure over too many years? Memories the subconscious holds onto even when

I am not consciously thinking about any of them? I genuinely do not know. What I know is that something shifted at some point without my permission and now my body responds differently to things it used to process without complaint.

Nobody told me that was going to happen. I am telling you now so it does not catch you off guard when it happens to you. And it probably will, in some form, in some way you are not expecting.

The stuff that sticks with you is not always dramatic. It is not always a death or a pediatric call or a mass casualty event. Sometimes it is a smell in a hallway. Sometimes it is a coroner's dirty glove. Sometimes it is four hours standing in the cold waiting for something you do not want to see but cannot leave until you do.

Develop your coping mechanisms early. Not after the cup is full. Before. We talk about what those look like in detail later in this book. What I want you to take from this chapter is simpler than that. Pay attention to what you are carrying. Not just the big calls but the small ones that add up. Not just the dramatic images but the sensory details that embed themselves somewhere below the level of conscious thought and resurface when you least expect them.

They are in there. And the sooner you acknowledge that, the better chance you have of managing them before they manage you.

Chapter 5: Burnout Starts Earlier Than You Think

Burnout does not announce itself. It does not show up one day with a clear message that you have reached your limit. It builds quietly, underneath everything else you are managing, and by the time most providers recognize it they are already well past the early signs they missed along the way.

It starts before your first shift. We talked in Chapter 1 about the gap between what you expect this career to look like and what it actually is. That gap is where burnout begins. You signed up for the dramatic calls. You are going to spend most of your career on the calls we talked about in Chapter 1, the ordinary ones, the lonely ones, the ones that never make it onto television. That is not a complaint about those calls. Those people deserve excellent care and you will provide it. But if you walk through the door expecting *Rescue 911* every shift, the daily reality of this job will start wearing on you long before you have the experience to recognize what is happening.

Add to that the financial reality. You will likely work two or three jobs to make ends meet. You will come to your shifts already tired. Your family and friends will not always understand why you cannot make it to dinner or why you need to sleep when everyone else is available.

Maybe this isn't news to you. But talking about it and facing it head-on will help you see the warning signs when they show up.

Here is what my warning signs looked like. I am sharing them because I missed all three of them until my cup had already started to overflow.

The first was my temper. I do not raise my voice with my staff. It does not help anyone and it is not who I am as a leader. During COVID I did it twice. The first time was with a crew member who was exhausted and angry because he kept getting assigned to COVID-potential calls while his full-time partner could not respond to those calls because we did not yet have PPE in the right size for him. He pushed back on a dispatch and said he was not going. I raised my voice. I told him he was right to feel that way and we would talk about it after the call. Then I told him, in terms I will leave to your imagination, to go take the job. The second time was a scene where our COVID protocols were being partially followed, but not fully. Both crew members were exposed in ways they should not have been. I raised my voice at both of them. Both apologized to me afterward for putting me in that position.

I am not proud of either moment. I understood why it happened. But the fact that it happened at all was a signal I did not stop to read.

The second warning sign was what I did with my time off. I was playing video games until three or four in the morning. Sleeping until noon. Not because I was tired, though I was. Because I was escaping. I did not want to be present in my own life. I did not want to sit still long enough to think about what I had been doing and seeing every day. The games were not a hobby. They were an exit door I kept walking through.

The third was the movies. I love *Star Wars*. I love *Patton*. I love *Saving Private Ryan*. Films I had watched a dozen times without much more than the normal emotional response. Suddenly I was crying at all of them. Not during the sad parts. Just crying. I did not understand why until I mentioned it to a colleague and he looked at me and said, "You need to talk to someone. Now."

It took me a few more years before I actually listened. That is a few more years I would take back if I could.

Now let me tell you about the hero identity trap, because I fell into it personally and I know what it costs.

I came into this career with a head full of *Rescue 911*. I wore the shirts. I had the mugs. I built part of my identity around being the person who ran toward the emergencies. And for a long time I did not see anything wrong with that. Then COVID came and the world decided that people like me were heroes whether we wanted the label or not.

I had a marked unit parked in front of my house. Every night the neighborhood came outside and clapped. And every night I stayed inside. I did not want to be recognized. I did not want the attention. I had people dying on my watch and a neighborhood applauding, and I could not reconcile those two things standing on my own front steps.

My neighbor came to talk to me about it one day. He was retired from public affairs in the United States Coast Guard. He had been to TWA Flight 800. He had been to September 11th. To Katrina. To the BP oil spill. He had stood at the edge of more disasters than most people will ever see in a lifetime. He told me I had to go outside even if I did not want to. That the people clapping were not doing it for me specifically. They were doing it for what I represented. And by staying inside I was taking that from them.

I went outside.

What he understood that I did not yet was that making any kind of emergency response career into your entire identity is dangerous in both directions. When things are good it inflates you in ways that are hard to sustain. When things are hard it has nowhere to put you except down. You are not a hero. You work in a profession that allows you to do some heroic things every once in a while. The rest of the time you are a person with a life and relationships and needs that have nothing to do with an ambulance. Protect that person. EMS is what you do. It is not who you are.

There is one proactive step I want to name specifically before we get to the hardest part of this chapter. Build your personal board of directors. That is not a corporate concept borrowed for effect. It is the most useful framework I know for the kind of support this career requires. Your personal board of directors is the small group of people you can call at any hour who will stop what they are doing and pick up. They will tell you the truth when you need to hear it. They will call you out when you are off track and do it without judgment. Some of them will be inside EMS and understand the world you are operating in. Some will be outside it entirely, and that outside perspective matters more than you think. Build that group intentionally and protect it. It will be the thing that catches you when the warning signs you missed have already stacked up.

There is one more thing I need to say plainly in this chapter and I am not going to soften it.

First responder suicide rates in this country exceed line of duty deaths from all other causes combined. More of us die by our own hand than in crashes, on scenes, or from exposure to illness. That is not a statistic that gets discussed enough in this profession and the silence around it costs lives.

The weight of this job accumulates. The calls, the missed holidays, the financial pressure, the physical toll, the things that stick with you that we talked about in Chapter 4. When people carry all of that without support, without coping mechanisms, without anyone checking in, the cup overflows in the worst possible way.

If you are struggling, say something. To your supervisor, your partner, your board of directors, a mental health professional, a crisis line. Saying something is not weakness. Staying silent until you cannot anymore is the thing that ends careers and ends lives.

Pay attention to your warning signs. Learn what they look like for you before you need that knowledge. And when you see them in someone else, say the same thing my colleague said to me.

You need to talk to someone. Now.

Chapter 6: Your Partner

Close to twenty years in this career and I have had more partners than I can count. Some I worked with once and never again. Others became part of the fabric of my life in ways I never saw coming. The guy who was standing next to me on my first shift? He was a groomsman at my wedding. Another supervisor I looked up to early in my career? Fifteen years later I became his boss. I have been to their weddings and their kids' birthdays. I have gotten the late-night phone calls and made them too. These are not coworkers in the way people outside this job understand the word. They are people who have seen you at your worst and stayed. That is the kind of bond that forms in EMS and nobody tells you about it before you start.

Your partner is not just the person sitting in the other seat of the rig. They are your coworker, your crew, sometimes your therapist, and occasionally your biggest headache. Get a good one and do everything you can to keep working with them. Not exclusively. You need to learn from different people and different styles. But when you find someone who clicks, protect that.

Here is what a truly good partner looks like in practice. You show up, you do your rig check, you get a call. And from the moment you walk through the door on that scene, you and your partner are moving. Nobody called a play. Nobody said "you take the airway, I'll get the AED." You just know. The crew might barely say a word out loud the entire call and yet everything is getting done in the right order at the right time. That is what a real partnership looks like. It is not magic. It is two people who have worked together long enough and trust each other enough that the job flows.

I learned some of my most important lessons not from training or textbooks but from watching the people I worked beside. Early in my career I worked with a supervisor who was ten or fifteen years older than me. On paper we had nothing in common. He liked baseball. I could not care less about baseball. I figured we would be cordial and that would be it. Then he started talking about *Star Wars* and that was the end of that assumption. But more important than what we talked about was what I watched him do. Every shift, every call, he had what he needed. Personal gear clipped to a utility belt, always within reach, added to over time as he figured out what he was missing. I watched that and it became a part of me. I still wear my version of that utility belt today. Other providers will tell you only new people do that. I have been doing this for two decades and I still have it on. Because that partner, without ever sitting me down and giving me a lesson, showed me what it looked like to always be prepared.

Not every partnership starts with that kind of natural chemistry. When I was working SCTU (Specialty Care Transport, interfacility calls with a registered nurse and two EMTs), my partner and I developed our own unofficial way of sizing up whoever was assigned as our third that shift. When we started the night we would play "Goodbye Horses". If you have ever seen *Silence of the Lambs*, you know the scene. (If you haven't, go look it up.) And we would start quoting Buffalo Bill. Every time. On purpose. If the third EMT went quiet and spent the rest of the shift staring at the floor, we knew it was going to be a long night. If they broke out laughing and jumped in, we knew they were going to be okay. It sounds ridiculous. It was ridiculous. But it worked. Because what we were really testing was whether this person could hang. Whether they had a sense of humor about the job. Whether they were going to be a real part of the crew or just occupy a seat.

That matters more than most people realize.

There's another "test" a coworker taught me, after he learned it training brand new cadets. After every call, ask yourself three questions. What went right? What went wrong? What can I do better? A good partner will do this with you honestly. They will not just tell you what you want to hear. They will give you real feedback and take real feedback in return. That habit, boring as it sounds, is one of the fastest ways to get better at this job. Most people don't do it because nobody told them to. Now I am telling you.

A bad partner is not just annoying. When you are new, a bad partner costs you learning time you will never get back. Every shift you spend with someone who is checked out, or who resists being guided, or who guides you in the wrong direction because they have been doing it wrong for years, is a shift where you are not growing. You are just surviving the hours.

And at its worst, a bad partner is a threat. To your patient. To you. In this situation, you protect your patients first, every call, no exceptions. You learn what you can, even if most of it is what not to do. You document honestly. And you talk to a supervisor you trust, not to complain but because a partner operating below the standard is a safety issue, and naming it is part of your job, not a betrayal of theirs.

You may not be able to choose your partner. You can always choose not to let their standard become yours. If you do not recognize that someone next to you is operating below the standard, you might not catch the thing that falls through the cracks on a serious call. That is not a hypothetical. That is the job.

You will learn something from every partner you ever have. Sometimes it is what to do. Sometimes it is exactly what not to do. Pay attention either way.

And if you find yourself on a shift with someone who laughs at the right moments, works without needing to be told, and tells you the truth after a tough call? Do not take that for granted. Those people are not easy to find.

Chapter 7: The System Will Frustrate You

At some point in your career, probably sooner than you expect, you are going to look around and think that the entire system is broken. You are not wrong. But understanding why it is the way it is, and learning how to operate inside it without losing your mind, is one of the most important skills you will ever develop in this profession.

Let's start at the hospital.

Most agencies have a difficult relationship with the ER they transport to most often. There are exceptions, usually when your crew shows up enough that the staff actually knows you and has seen what you can do. But in a lot of cases, you are going to walk in with a patient and feel like you are invisible. Nurses are busy. There are not enough beds. In some parts of the country you spend thirty minutes at the hospital, patient on your stretcher, waiting for a bed to open up. In others you are waiting hours. And sometimes it feels like the hospital staff looks at you as the person who brought them more work, not the person who kept that patient alive long enough to get there.

Here is something nobody teaches you in school: how to give a good report. I have watched

EMTs get torn apart by charge nurses for giving a slow, unfocused rundown that buried the important information under a pile of things nobody needed to know at that moment. Learn this early. The nurse does not care about the hip surgery from twelve years ago when your patient is presenting with chest pain. What they want is the last set of vitals, what the patient called you for, what your clinical impression is, and anything else that is actually relevant. Clear and concise. That is the game. Once you learn how to walk in and give a sharp report, the dynamic with hospital staff starts to shift. Respect is earned in this profession and the ER is no different.

Now let's talk about dispatch.

Radios do not work when they should. You will get sent to the wrong address. Dispatch will sometimes try to tell you what to do when the information flow should really be going the other direction. There will be moments when you are frustrated and that frustration is going to want to come out of your mouth on the radio.

I learned this the hard way. I was a supervisor (experienced enough to know better) when dispatch called down asking if I had any ambulances available. I told them (and I am not proud of this), "You are the dispatch center. You tell me." They responded with "way to be helpful" and hung up.

They were right.

About an hour later, after things had quieted down, I called dispatch and apologized. Because when I actually thought about it, dispatch is sitting there handling every 911 call coming into your coverage area simultaneously. They are on the line with a caller, they are sending you and police and fire, and another call is already coming in behind it. They are underpaid and overworked just like we are. Losing track of whether a truck is clear or not in the middle of all of that is not incompetence. It is what happens when you are a few people managing an entire system in real time.

Remember that the next time you want to say something you cannot take back on the radio.

Protocols are their own source of frustration. You will encounter moments where following the protocol feels like it is getting in the way of what the patient actually needs. I understand that feeling. But I want you to think about protocols the way I do, which is a lot like the way I think about OSHA rules. They are written in blood. Something happened, or something nearly happened, that the system was trying to make sure could not happen again. They exist for a reason. Respect them even when they feel limiting. And if you truly believe a protocol is wrong, the right move is to raise it through the proper channels, not to quietly ignore it on scene.

The frustration that lives inside your own agency is a different beast entirely.

If you are starting at a volunteer agency, prepare yourself for the reality that leadership is sometimes decided by popularity contest. Elections happen. And it does not always matter who has the better ideas or the stronger qualifications. What matters is who has the most friends in the room that night. Find a volunteer agency with the same elected leadership for thirty or forty years and you have found an agency that is probably doing things the same way they did them thirty or forty years ago. There are exceptions to everything, but that is the pattern.

And whether you are at a volunteer agency or a paid one, there is a very good chance that the person supervising you got that role because they were a good clinician. Not because anyone assessed whether they could actually manage people, navigate a budget, or handle the kind of complex human situations that come with leadership. We promote our best providers and then cross our fingers. Sometimes it works out. Often it does not. Your supervisor may be learning how to supervise at the same time you are learning how to be an EMT. Be patient with that even when it is hard.

Here is what I want you to take from all of this:

It may feel hopeless sometimes. It may feel tedious. But a lot of what frustrates you is happening for a reason, even if that reason is not immediately obvious. The job is to understand the system well enough to work inside it, and eventually, to make it better.

You have two options when something is wrong. You try to change it from within. Or you vote with your feet and leave. People do not leave agencies over pay as often as they claim. They leave over culture. They leave over leadership. I know agencies that pay significantly more than mine and they are always posting open positions. Mine has a wait list. That difference is not about the paycheck.

I lived this myself. I was at a point in my career where I could see the changes that needed to be made and I also knew that a merger that was taking place, and I was not going to have a job on the other side of it. Years before, I had sat in an interview for the top position at that organization and told them directly: "This is my passion, this is what I want to do in life. I will do it and either it will be here or it will be somewhere else, but it would be a mistake for the organization if it isn't here."

It wasn't there.

I left and went somewhere else. I have two awards on my wall now to show for it.

Be the change you want for this profession. But do it intelligently and sustainably. Not because you think you know better than everyone around you, but because you have put in the work to actually understand what better looks like. I started in EMS at nineteen years old and by twenty I was already sure I should be running the place. That was foolish. I eventually got a leadership role I was not ready for. Some of the decisions I made in that role were the right calls. I just was not mature enough yet to deliver them the right way, and I regret that. There are other decisions I genuinely wish I had not made at all. Both of those things shaped me into the leader I am today.

The system is frustrating. It has always been frustrating. The people who last in this profession are the ones who learn to navigate that frustration instead of being consumed by it.

Chapter 8: Your Body Is Going to Take a Hit

Nobody in your EMT class is going to spend much time on this. They will teach you proper lifting techniques and tell you to get enough sleep and leave it at that. What they will not tell you is that this career will work on your body in ways that accumulate slowly over years until one day you notice the damage that has already been done. Start paying attention now, before that day comes.

Let's start with sleep, because it will affect everything else.

I have always been a night owl, so the overnight shifts never hit me as hard as they hit some people. But there is a real difference between being a night owl and being genuinely sleep deprived, and this career will introduce you to the second one whether you are ready for it or not. The 911 caller does not care that you just finished your sixth call in a row. Dispatch does not care that you have been running all night and were supposed to get off twenty minutes ago. There is another call and you are going to take it.

Have you ever been so exhausted while driving to an emergency that you were clenching the muscles in your leg just to feel awake? I have. More than once. That is not a sustainable or safe way to operate, and yet it became a pattern. That is the reality of this job.

The data on this is not subtle. Shift work and overnight hours will take years off your life. Your body is not designed to sleep while everyone around you is awake and functioning. Blackout curtains and white noise become necessities, not luxuries. Your agency will tell you to get eight hours of rest before a shift. Your agency will also not pay you enough to live on without working multiple jobs, which means the eight hour requirement and the financial reality of your life are going to be in direct conflict regularly.

The longest stretch I ever worked between two agencies was forty-eight hours straight. It should not have happened. It was not safe. And it is not an unusual story in this industry. If anything, it is closer to the norm than anyone in leadership wants to admit. Maybe you will be part of the generation that changes that. I hope so.

Now let's talk about your body.

In New Jersey, the benchmark is that each EMT should be able to lift one hundred and fifty pounds, the logic being that a crew of two should be able to handle a three hundred pound patient. What that standard does not account for is that your partner may be significantly shorter or taller than you, or that one of you is coming off a double shift, or that your patient is not three hundred pounds, they are four hundred and fifty pounds and there is no additional help available.

School will teach you proper lifting and moving technique. What school cannot fully prepare you for is the patient who is wedged between the toilet and the wall with no room to approach them correctly. Or the narrow staircase in a hundred-year-old house. Or the fact that sometimes there is simply no good way to do it and you are going to lift awkwardly and hope for the best.

I can remember clearly the first time I tweaked my back. It was not a dramatic call. I was helping move a patient down one step from a house to the ambulance. The patient was not unusually heavy. I was not even supposed to be there that day. I had some time before work, heard the call go out for a structure fire as a volunteer, and decided to stop in. I did everything right technically. That one tweak turned into fifteen years of on-and-off back pain that I manage with over the counter medication, a chiropractor, and exercise. One step. One moment.

It will not always be dramatic when it happens. That is the point.

Diet is its own challenge and it is more connected to your mental health than most people realize.

I am fortunate to live in New Jersey where twenty-four hour diners exist and you can get a real meal at three in the morning if you have the time to sit down. But after working a bad call, do you really think you are reaching for the grilled chicken? There is a reason comfort food exists and there is a reason you will eat it. The problem is when that becomes the default every shift.

What happens when you do not have time to sit down at all? When all you have access to is the microwave at a convenience store or the snack room at the hospital? The frozen breakfast sandwiches and the chips and the cookies disappear immediately from that hospital snack room. The fresh fruit sits there until someone throws it out. You will run on caffeine. Many providers add nicotine to that rotation, and I am telling you to avoid it but will also tell you the truth about my own record on this.

I had finally gotten my cigarette habit under control. An occasional one when the stress got to be too much, but mostly done with it. Then I deployed to Hurricane Helene in North Carolina for my first FEMA Urban Search and Rescue deployment. That was almost two years ago. I have been using nicotine pouches ever since. I am not proud of it. I am telling you anyway because this book is not about pretending the job does not get to you. It does. And sometimes it gets to you in ways you did not see coming before you were already in the middle of them.

Here is the bigger picture that I want you to sit with:

You will not be able to do this forever. Not at full intensity. Your body will accumulate wear. Your mental health will be tested in ways that have physical consequences. The providers who make it to the end of a long career with their health reasonably intact are the ones who started thinking about this early, not the ones who figured it out after the damage was already done.

Start thinking about your exit strategy early. Not with the mindset that you'll be giving up, but because you need to be realistic. The career will not wait for you to figure it out.

Prioritize your mental health first and the physical stuff tends to follow. When you are in a good place mentally you make better choices about food, about exercise, about the things you reach for when a bad call stays with you. Meal prep when you can. Move your body consistently, not just when you feel like it. Use the tools available to you, including medical ones, when you need help. And when your favorite partner suggests splitting a crave case from White Castle at two in the morning after a rough night, sometimes the answer has to be no.

Your body is the only equipment you cannot replace. Treat it accordingly.

Chapter 9: This Job Can Kill You

I want to say something that does not get said plainly enough in this profession.

This job can kill you.

Not burn you out. Not wear you down. Not send you home exhausted. Kill you. And if you are going to do this work with clear eyes, you need to understand that before you ever step foot on an ambulance.

There are four ways it happens most often.

The first is the vehicle itself. Lights and sirens driving is one of the most dangerous things you will do in this career. Every time you are behind the wheel of an ambulance running lights and sirens, you are navigating intersections where other drivers may not hear you, may not see you, or may panic and make the wrong decision when they do. Providers die in crashes. Patients die in crashes. It happens more than the public realizes and it happens to experienced crews who did everything right. This is why our industry is actively pushing to reduce the number of lights and sirens responses. Not every call warrants them and the data shows that the risk does not always match the benefit. Learn your agency's protocols on this early and take them seriously.

The second is the scene itself. You will respond to calls where the danger is not the patient but the environment around them. Unstable structures. Violence. Fires. Active situations that have not been fully controlled before you arrive. Scene safety is not a box you check on your way through the door. It is a continuous assessment from the moment you pull up until the moment you leave. The patient in front of you cannot be helped if you become a patient yourself.

I was operating as EMS Branch Commander at a large fire when the second floor collapsed onto the first. Nobody was in immediate danger, but I looked over and noticed two crew members from another agency standing nearby without their helmets on. I pulled them aside. I told them there is a reason every policy at every EMS agency in this country requires a helmet at a fire scene. Then I told them to go put their helmets on. They did not work for me. We were from different agencies entirely. But as EMS Branch I was responsible for every EMS provider on that scene and I was not going to watch someone put themselves at risk because they decided the policy did not apply to them that day. Wear your gear. Every time. The policy exists because someone learned that lesson the hard way before you arrived.

The third is sleep deprivation. We talked about this in the body chapter and it belongs here too, because it is not just a health issue. It is a safety issue. Driving an ambulance after a full overnight of back-to-back calls, or worse, after working a shift at your second job before coming in, is impaired driving. The research on sleep deprivation consistently shows that operating a vehicle on no sleep is comparable to operating one drunk. You already read about clenching your leg muscles just to feel awake behind the wheel. That is not an unusual story in this profession. Providers fall asleep at the wheel. It happens on the way to calls. It happens on the way home. It has killed people. If you are at the point where you genuinely cannot keep your eyes open, say something to your partner or your supervisor. There is no version of that conversation that ends worse than the alternative.

The fourth is exposure. What you cannot see can kill you just as surely as anything else.

In New Jersey alone, we lost more EMS providers to COVID-19 than were lost on September 11th. I want you to sit with that number for a moment. More. A virus that nobody fully understood yet moved through our ranks while we kept showing up because there was no one else to go. We did not stop. We could not stop. That is who we are as a profession. But the cost was real and it was paid in lives.

I went to the 9/11 Memorial Museum in New York City not long ago. I was moving through the exhibits and I stopped in front of a shield. A badge belonging to a Port Authority Police Officer. The last name on it was Mazza. No relation to me, as far as I know. But I stood there and I felt it anyway. A name that looked like mine on a badge behind glass in a museum dedicated to people who went to work one morning and did not come home. It made something abstract suddenly very concrete.

I knew a provider from my SCTU days, not well, but enough. We overlapped at the same company. We had talked more than once about cigars, the way you bond over something small with someone you see regularly without ever becoming close. He died early in COVID. He was not a stranger. He was someone I had stood next to, someone I had exchanged a few words with, someone I knew. And then he was gone.

That is what this looks like up close. Not a statistic. A person you know, or almost knew, who is no longer here.

I am not telling you this to frighten you away from the job. I am telling you because you deserve to know what you are signing up for in full. Wear your PPE every time without exception. Take scene safety seriously even when the call sounds routine. Drive that ambulance with the weight of what you are carrying in mind. And understand that the providers who came before you paid a price for this profession that most of the public will never know or fully appreciate.

Honor that by coming home.

Chapter 10: Documentation and the Unglamorous Admin Side

Nobody gets into EMS because they love paperwork. If that is why you are here, I have serious concerns about your life choices. But documentation is one of those things that will define your career in ways that have nothing to do with how good you are on scene, and the providers who treat it as an afterthought eventually find that out the hard way.

Let me start at the beginning.

Growing up I was always told my handwriting was fit for a doctor or a lawyer and nothing else. Which made it quietly hilarious that I entered a field where, at the time, handwritten charts were the only option. Some providers wrote in cursive. I printed because I wanted someone to actually be able to read it. What I was not prepared for was that EMT school barely touched on how to actually write a Patient Care Report. Fortunately I was volunteering at the time, and my supervisors sat me down and walked me through it.

I cringe looking back at those early charts. They are technically complete in the sense that information is present. But they do not paint a picture. They do not tell the story of the call. I know now how to write a narrative that puts the reader on scene with me, that documents not just what I found but why I made the decisions I made. That skill took years to develop and nobody handed it to me on day one. I am handing it to you now. The goal of a PCR narrative is not to fill a box. It is to paint a picture so clear that someone who was never on that call can understand exactly what happened and why.

This matters more than most new providers realize.

In 2019 I was called to testify about a call. The chart in question was from 2009 or 2010. Nearly a decade earlier. The agency I worked for at the time could not even locate a copy of it at first. Think about that. How was I supposed to testify truthfully under oath about a call I went on ten years prior, without a chart, when I had been on hundreds if not thousands of calls between that day and the day I was sitting in that room? The chart was eventually found. I read it and cringed at how much my documentation had evolved. Fortunately I have a strange memory and the call had stuck with me because it was high profile enough that someone had photographed me working it. I was prepared to testify. The case settled before I ever got the chance.

But here is the lesson: You are going to write a chart today and you are going to think that nobody will ever look at it again. You might be right. You might also be sitting across from an attorney in five years trying to reconstruct a call from memory with nothing to work from. Write every chart as if that is where it is going. Because sometimes it is.

Another administrative aspect of the job that does not get discussed enough is money, which touches everything.

Most agencies bill for their services. That bill is how the agency gets paid, which is how the lights stay on and how your paycheck gets cut. If your chart is incomplete, if the documentation does not support the level of care that was provided, the agency does not get reimbursed. Or they get reimbursed at a lower rate than the call warranted. We have conversations in this industry about pay parity and living wages and why EMS providers are underpaid. Part of that conversation has to include the fact that poor documentation means agencies are leaving money on the table that was already earned. You cannot advocate for better pay while handing in charts that get the call denied. These things are connected.

Now let's talk about the reality of documenting in the field.

Everything has moved digital. Toughbooks, tablets, electronic patient care reporting systems. That is the world you are entering. But experienced providers will tell you that paper never fully goes away and they are right. I keep a notebook. Most providers I respect keep a notebook. On a chaotic call you jot down your key findings, your interventions, your times, your vitals. The important information that you absolutely cannot afford to reconstruct from memory when you finally sit down to chart. Less experienced providers skip this and hug the tablet instead, trying to document in real time while also managing a patient. That is a recipe for gaps.

Here is my honest and completely anecdotal theory about why EMS providers resist documentation as a group. I think this field attracts people with a certain personality type that gravitates toward the new and changing. We love new things. We love the pace. We love the fact that every hour can look completely different from the last. Documentation is the opposite of all of that. It is repetitive, it requires sustained focus, and the feedback loop is slow. It makes sense that the people who thrive on scene are often the same people who struggle to sit still long enough to chart properly afterward. I am not a researcher but I think that dynamic deserves serious study.

The digital shift has made some things better and some things worse. The upside is that thorough documentation is more possible than ever. Better records mean better continuity of care for patients down the line. The downside is that we used to physically leave a copy of the paper chart at the hospital before we left the ER.

That built in a natural deadline. Now there is no automatic handoff. Do not be the crew that has to be chased down to complete their charts.

What I want you to take from this chapter is that documentation is not the unglamorous part of the job that you tolerate in between the real work. It is part of the real work. Master it the same way you master your clinical skills. Develop a consistent process, write with the same thoroughness every single time regardless of how tired you are or how straightforward the call seemed, and do it in a timely fashion. Your patients deserve an accurate record of their care. Your agency depends on it financially. And someday, sitting with a lawyer in a room you cannot currently imagine, you might be very glad you took it seriously.

Chapter 11: Dealing With Death

My father used to read the obituaries first thing every morning. When I asked him why, he would say he was checking to see if he had died. He passed on Father's Day in 2013 after a year-long fight with cancer. I think about that joke more than he probably ever intended me to. Only two things are guaranteed from the moment you are born: death and taxes. He was not wrong. This career will put you closer to the first one than most people ever get.

Let's talk about it.

I was nineteen years old on my second shift, second call, when I watched someone die for the first time. A woman, around forty, with a husband and two kids who were in the room screaming for us to save their mother, their wife, their everything. What I have never told anyone outside of this profession is what happened after.

I had no real role on that call. I had basic CPR training and nothing else. My job was to get equipment for the actual EMTs, both of whom I mentioned in an earlier chapter, one of whom would later stand at my wedding and the other who I would eventually become supervisor to. When we got back and cleaned up the ambulance I must have been visibly somewhere else. It was after three in the morning when we caught the call and by the time we were done it was nearly six and the shift was ending. Whether I looked the way I did because of the hour or because I had just watched a person die, I honestly cannot tell you. Probably both.

My colleague, the one who I would eventually become supervisor to, put his arm around my shoulders and said, "you can't save them all." Then he told an off-color joke about the whole thing. I paused. I looked at him. I cracked a smile and laughed softly. That is how I got home.

I was nineteen. I had class afterward. I went to the commuter lounge at Seton Hall and my best friend since grammar school and a few others came and sat with me. They could tell I was off. They wanted the details, the way people always do when they find out you work in EMS. I just shook my head and said I watched someone die today. Not much to tell. I barely ate. I sat there wondering if I had made the right choice. But I kept coming back to that joke. That stupid, off-color, perfect joke. It is what got me through that day.

After a few days it started to feel normal. By the time my next shift came around—a week later, since that was my rotation as a volunteer back then—I was excited to go back and learn more. That is what surprised me most. That it became something I could carry and still keep moving.

It took me years to learn that the traumatic deaths, the violent and unexpected ones, stick with you differently than others. They flash before your eyes when you are near the place where it happened. That tends to fade over months, sometimes years. During COVID I saw so much death that it all melted together into something I can barely separate into individual memories. I do not know if that is coping or numbness or both. Maybe there is not much difference between the two after a while. What's another corpse?

That is a dark thing to say. I am saying it anyway because if you stay in this career long enough you may find yourself thinking something similar, and I want you to know that is a signal worth paying attention to, not something to be ashamed of. That is your signal to talk to someone because your cup is about to overflow. Then there are the children.

Children are their own category.

I have been fortunate not to have many critical pediatric calls in my career. I know providers who had done this job for twenty years, seen everything, and then lost a child on a call and walked out of the profession weeks later. Their cup overflowed. When I respond to a pediatric call, I go back to something deeper than training. I believe that if it is someone's time, nothing we do can fully change that. My faith has shifted considerably over the years, but I hold onto the belief that sometimes the outcome is simply beyond us, that we are not the final word on who lives and who dies. What I can control is the quality of care I provide and the resilience I bring to the scene. The rest I leave where I have to leave it.

There is a distinction worth making between arriving to find someone already gone, and watching someone die while you are working them. I never fully considered it until I sat down to write this. A body in full rigor is a different thing than a person. Lividity changes the color of the skin. The smell is unlike anything else. You can compartmentalize more easily when the person died long before you were called and there was never anything to be done. It is harder when you are doing chest compressions and you feel the moment the fight is over.

When it is done and the call is over, nobody speaks right away. The crew moves like robots. They clean the truck. They restock the equipment. They get back in service. They are resetting themselves the only way they know how. If you are lucky, your supervisor is there and they are checking on you. If the call was high-profile enough, an officer involved shooting, a child, something that makes the news, there may be a formal debrief, grief counseling if the agency has it set up, maybe time off. But that is the exception. The standard is you clean the truck, you restock, and you go back to work. The world does not stop because you just watched someone die and neither does the radio. If you are less lucky, someone else has already called 911 while you were cleaning up and you are being dispatched to a dementia patient or a broken arm or a toothache before you have had a single minute to process what just happened.

I am not sure how anyone reconciles that. I have been doing this for close to twenty years and I still do not have a clean answer for it. You go back to your coping mechanisms. You go back to the things that keep you grounded. And you keep going.

But here's the thing I didn't expect: the deaths are not what stay with me the most anymore. I most remember the saves.

It was twelve thirty in the morning when we got called. On the way there, my gut told me she was just sound asleep, that this was going to be one of *those* calls. She was too young to really be having an MI.

She was in full cardiac arrest when we arrived. A "widow-maker" heart attack. We did CPR, used the AED; the paramedics arrived and ran their ACLS protocol, and we brought her back.

About a year later I was at a car show, and a woman walked up to me and hugged me. It took me a moment to place her. She was the woman from that call. Standing in front of me in the sunlight at a car show, alive, because we had been there that night.

That is what stays with me now more than anything.

But honestly, those moments may be rare. They may never come for you in the way they came for me. Until they do, or if they don't, the deaths may be what you carry. That is real and it is valid and it does not mean you are doing something wrong. Understand this before your first death:

Nothing you do will change the fact that it is coming. Death comes for all of us from the moment we are born. My father knew that and found a way to joke about it every morning over the obituaries. Knowing that, really internalizing it, takes away the mythology of racing the reaper or saving lives and replaces it with something more honest. Your job is emergency medicine. You cannot change every outcome. Some of the people you respond to are going to die and there is nothing you could have done differently.

That is not failure. That is the job.

What you can do is show up, provide the best care you are capable of, and be present for the worst moment of someone's life. Sometimes that is enough to bring someone back. Sometimes it is enough to make sure they did not die alone. Both of those things matter.

The joke my colleague told me at the end of my second shift does not hold up in polite company. I am not going to repeat it here. But it kept me in this profession for twenty years and counting. Find your version of it. And hold onto it.

Chapter 12: When Patients Are Awful to You

I have been overweight my entire life. I have been called fat my entire life. Long before I ever put on a uniform, I had already spent years learning how to let an insult land somewhere that did not stop me. That is armor. I built mine early, without choosing to, and I still told myself it fit better than it did. I am telling you this because that armor is exactly what this career is going to test, and the way you handle being treated badly by the people you are trying to help says a lot about who you are as a provider. You may build your armor on the job. I had a head start. Either way, you are going to need it. There's one call that has stayed with me for many years, even though the insult was not directed at me.

I was working a discharge transport to a nursing home with a partner who is a person of color. Our patient had dementia. On the way to the nursing home, he started calling my partner the N word. Repeatedly. I immediately told my partner to take the wheel and I would ride in the back for this leg of the trip. That was supposed to be his job on this shift. He refused. He looked at me and said the old man did not know what he was saying. That there was no real hate there because he was not really there. I pushed back.

He would not move. It was an uncomfortable ride to that nursing home. We laughed about it a lot afterward.

I want you to think about what my partner did on that call. He made a choice in real time that I was not capable of making for him. He assessed the situation, separated the behavior from the person, and kept working. That does not mean what was said was acceptable. It means he was a professional operating in a complicated moment. Not everyone could have done that. Not everyone should have to.

I want to say something plainly because our industry does not say it enough.

Being assaulted is not part of this job. I want to say that again. Being assaulted is not part of this job. Poor leaders will tell you it is. They will tell you to suck it up, that it comes with the territory, that this is what you signed up for. If you encounter that kind of leadership, it should go on your list of reasons to find somewhere better to work.

Will patients in medical crisis do things they would never do otherwise? Absolutely. A patient with low blood sugar, a head injury, a psychiatric episode—they may swing at you or spit at you or say things that would be unforgivable in any other context. In many of those cases, pressing charges is neither appropriate nor productive. But that line is not as blurry as our industry pretends it is, and the fact that we have let it get blurry is one of my genuine frustrations with this profession.

Here is the contrast that illustrates it best.

April 2020. COVID is in full swing. We had a local patient, chronically intoxicated, always a problem, who had apparently moved on to something harder. He was seeing thousands of Chucky dolls, the one from the movie, telling him to kill people. He needed treatment. Before we could get him secured he was out of the ambulance and heading toward traffic. I was there with law enforcement trying to stop him. He pushed me. One hand, contact on my chest, barely more than a graze. Six officers went on top of him immediately. We got him secured on the stretcher and the sergeant told me they would follow us to the hospital. I slammed the ambulance doors and told him, "No. Do your job and charge him with aggravated assault." He was taken aback. They reviewed the body camera footage, confirmed the contact, and he was charged. He served no time that I know of. Prisons are overcrowded. But the charge was filed and that mattered.

The year before that, a dementia patient kicked me in the testicles while we were trying to secure him to the cot. When I could breathe again and the officers asked if I was okay I laughed and said, "Yeah, what can you do, the guy is not there." Same instinct my partner had with the nursing home patient. The behavior was real. The person behind it was not.

In my mind the line was simple. The first patient I described had a long history of getting intoxicated and then turning combative. He made that choice, daily, and it was a choice that put myself, my partner, law enforcement officers, and the general public in danger. The dementia patient had no choice in his action. His disease took the wheel and there was no version of him underneath his disease that knew my testicles from a doorknob. One of them was a person who chose a path that led to harm. The other was a body running on a disease with nobody home to answer for it. That is the difference between accountability and understanding, and you will have to make that call in real time, often in seconds, with incomplete information.

Knowing the difference between those two calls, knowing when the situation calls for accountability and when it calls for understanding, is one of the more important judgment calls you will develop in this career. But never let anyone convince you that the answer is always just to absorb it and move on.

People will also criticize things that have nothing to do with the medical treatment itself. They will tell you that you took too long to get there. That the ride was too bumpy. That you should have done something differently. Most of that is noise. They are having the worst day of their life and you walked into the middle of it. They do not know your world any more than you know theirs. Let the noise be noise. Keep your head down and do your job. But know the difference between noise and genuine hate, and do not let anyone tell you those two things are the same.

You have the right to protect yourself and to press charges if you are assaulted. Full stop. Take a Defensive Tactics for EMS course if one is available to you. This is specific training designed for our environment, and the instructors who teach it can testify on your behalf if you ever need to demonstrate in court that you used their techniques correctly. Learn verbal de-escalation. Learn how to read a scene before it turns physical. And if your agency has ballistic protective equipment available, learn how to use it and when to wear it.

Some providers wear body armor on every shift and get mocked for it. They should not be mocked. If wearing it makes someone feel safer, that is a legitimate choice. It is personal protective equipment, the same as gloves or a mask. It exists to protect you and nothing else. It is not a force field and it is not an excuse to be reckless or aggressive. But if someone wants to wear it every day, that is their call to make. The thing that bothers me most about this whole piece of the job is not any individual patient or any single call. It is that our own industry does not take this seriously enough. If someone puts a hand on a police officer or a firefighter there is a swift and clear response. When it happens to us the default reaction is too often a shrug. We deserve better than that. You deserve better than that. And until the people running this industry start treating assaults on EMS providers the way they treat assaults on anyone else in public safety, keep advocating for yourself, because not enough people above you will do it for you.

Chapter 13: Your First Leadership Moment

There is a quote attributed to General Patton that I have carried with me for most of my career. “Lead me, follow me, or get out of my way.” I did not always understand what that meant. Learning it was a decade-long journey that taught me what it meant to lead in different situations and contexts.

I started volunteering in September of 2006 at nineteen years old. I did not have my EMT card yet, because college made it hard to get to EMT school right away. I *did* have enough maturity that the people around me noticed, and they put me to work. They taught me to drive the ambulance early. Lights and sirens, always to the hospital, never to a scene. It was the fun part and I knew it. When I finally got my EMT card in August of 2007, one of my instructors offered me my first paid EMS job on the spot. I took it. I thought I was ready for anything.

My supervisor at the volunteer agency had other ideas. He told me I was not ready to operate independently. I was annoyed. I was working paid shifts at a municipal agency. What did he mean I was not ready? A few months later he let me take my test to operate on my own, which at our agency meant you could bring an ambulance to a scene and potentially be the only medical provider there until a crew arrived. The person who administered my test was someone I call a friend today, a cop in town I had worked alongside enough times to trust.

He looked at me and said: "Do you know where all the things are?"

I said yes.

"Good. Because if you don't, you are going to look like an asshole."

"Do you know how to treat everyone?"

I said yes.

"Good. Because if you don't, you are going to look like an even bigger asshole. And get sued."

That was it. That was my test. He was handing me ownership and he knew it. It was empowering and terrifying in equal measure. I went home and studied anyway, not because I had to but because I did not want to look like an asshole. That is what accountability feels like when it is done right. He did not micromanage me into competence. He trusted me into it.

Not long after that test I was on a cardiac arrest—my first as a fully certified EMT, though not my first cardiac arrest overall. The crew chief stepped away to speak with the family and left me standing there with two EMTs who were newer than I was. No instruction. No handoff. Just the expectation that I would handle it.

I directed the call while also doing CPR. The three of us ran like a well-oiled machine even though we barely knew each other. When it was over I remember thinking that I liked this. I liked being the one making the calls. I liked the clarity of it.

What I did not yet understand was the difference between leading a call and leading people.

Being a good provider does not make you a good leader. The skills overlap in places, but they are not the same thing. On a call you are responsible for one patient at a time. As a leader you are responsible for the health, safety, and well-being of your patient, your crew, and everyone else on that scene simultaneously. The juggling act is larger. The stakes are distributed differently. And the feedback is slower, which means you can be doing it wrong for a long time before you find out.

I found out when they made me an Assistant Crew Chief at the volunteer agency. Everyone more experienced than me had moved on, and I was the most senior person left. They gave me the number two position, but there was no number one above me. At the time I felt snubbed. I felt like they did not trust me with the title I had earned. I was young and angry about it and I carried that chip visibly.

Looking back, they were doing me a favor. They knew I was the defacto leader by default. They also knew I was not truly ready for the full weight of it. They were trying to tell me something and I was not mature enough to hear it.

Leading on a call and leading an incident are also different animals. The clearest picture I have of what street level leadership actually looks like came a couple of years into my time as a supervisor. A heat wave knocked out power to two six-story buildings in town, both of them filled almost entirely with senior citizens, many of whom were handicapped or on oxygen. No working elevators. Emergency lighting so faint it barely counted. The paid fire department was on scene but not taking charge, even though they were supposed to be in charge of emergency management, which left me and two police officers to run the whole operation.

I was twenty-three years old and not getting paid for my time.

I drew on my Incident Command training and we built a plan. Systematic floor by floor search, prioritizing the oxygen-dependent patients first, then the handicapped residents, working outward from there. I coordinated the search, tracked the information, communicated with the officers, and kept the whole thing moving. It started just before eleven at night and we were not done until three in the morning.

That was the first time I understood what the Patton quote actually meant. The fire department was on scene and chose not to take charge. They were not going to lead. So the choice in front of me was the one Patton described: Lead, follow, or get out of the way. Nobody was leading, and people on oxygen were sitting in the dark on the sixth floor. Someone had to take control. That night I learned Patton's quote is not a threat you say to other people. It is a question the situation asks you, and you answer it by what you do next. At that incident, I chose to lead.

I say this with some humor, but mostly seriously: Be careful about how fast you chase the next title.

If what you love about this job is the medicine, if you genuinely love showing up on someone's worst day and making a difference, understand what you are trading away when you move up. I was talking with someone recently and mentioned offhandedly that I would have trouble moving to another state because I am only an EMT. They stopped me. They looked at me and said, "You are not an EMT anymore. Yes, you have your card. Yes, you keep your skills current. But you are not an EMT. You are a leader. Your job now is to make it possible for other people to do theirs."

They were right and it stung a little.

I still have my card. I still keep my skills sharp. But the reality of what I do every day is spreadsheets and budgets and policies and personnel decisions and conversations that have nothing to do with a patient in front of me. I sincerely miss treating patients. That is not a complaint. It is a truth I want you to have before you decide how fast to climb.

Your first leadership moment is coming. It may be on a call where someone steps back and everyone looks at you. It may be the first time you have to tell a newer provider they did something wrong. It may be managing a scene that is bigger and messier than anything you trained for. When it comes, fall back on what you know, trust the people around you, and do not let the size of the moment convince you that you need to perform instead of just lead.

The goal is not to look like you are in charge. The goal is to actually be in charge. There is a difference and people can always tell.

Chapter 14: How to Actually Survive This Job

To mis-quote *GI Joe*, knowing is *only* half the battle.

You have read a lot of hard truths in this book. You know what the job actually looks like. You know what it asks of your body, your relationships, your mental health, and your sense of self. You know the warning signs of burnout and what happens when people carry too much without support. Knowing all of that is genuinely valuable. It is also not enough on its own.

This chapter is about the other half. The daily decisions and habits that determine whether you are still standing at the end of a long career or whether the job has ground you down before you ever got there.

Let's start with the coping mechanisms, because the wrong ones are everywhere and easy to reach.

Alcohol. Nicotine. Stimulants. Gambling. They are all available, they all work in the short term, and they will all cost you more than they give you over time. I know this because I have watched it happen to people and because I have had my own versions of reaching for the wrong thing when the pressure got high enough. I mentioned the nicotine pouches in Chapter 8. I am not proud of it.

The right coping mechanisms are less immediately satisfying and require more effort to maintain. Exercise is the one I hear most often, and I will be honest with you about my own relationship with it. I have always been overweight. Exercise hurts quickly when you are carrying extra weight and the results do not come fast enough to sustain motivation when you are already tired from the job. I do not know how much of that has been legitimate pain and how much of it has been a convenient story I told myself to avoid doing the hard thing. Probably some of both. What I do know is that good exercise, being outside, walking, moving your body in whatever way you can sustain, genuinely helps. Not because it solves anything but because it gives the stress somewhere to go that is not your body, slowly breaking down from the inside.

Find what works for you and commit to it. For me it has been reading, the occasional video game, and a good cigar on a quiet evening. Simple things that require me to be present and not thinking about work. The key phrase is *not thinking about work*. Whatever your version of that is, protect it.

Vacations and breaks are not optional. I do not roll over PTO for my staff, and the primary reason is not financial. I want them to actually leave. To decompress. To go somewhere that is not this. People think that taking a trip and seeing new things is the same as a vacation, and for some people it is. For me, a trip is an experience, interesting and worthwhile, but it does not turn everything off the way sitting on a beach does. There is a difference between stimulating your mind with new things and genuinely resting it. Know which one you need and make sure you are getting that, not just the experience that is easier to explain to other people.

Your mind will tell you when it needs a break if you are paying attention. Listen to it before it starts saying it louder.

And if a beach is not in the budget (and for a lot of us in this profession it is not), the principle still holds. Rest is not about the destination. It is about genuinely turning the job off. A day with your phone in another room. A morning you do not set an alarm. A walk with no destination. The providers who burn out are not the ones who could not afford Hawaii. They are the ones who never gave their minds permission to stop, whatever stopping looks like for them. Find the version you can afford and take it as seriously as you would take a call.

If I could go back, this is what I would tell my nineteen-year-old self, standing on the front steps in that oversized coat, who thought he already knew most of what he needed to know.

Lean into the fact that this is the real world and not *Rescue 911*. The sooner you make peace with the gap between those two things, the sooner you can start doing the actual job instead of mourning the one you imagined. Prioritize your health early. Your eating habits, your sleep, your exercise. The choices you make in your first years in this career will compound in both directions. Good habits compound into a body and a mind that can sustain decades of this work. Bad ones compound into the back pain and the burnout and the reaching for the wrong things when the pressure gets high enough.

And listen to the people who have been doing this longer than you. When someone more experienced tells you that you have a lot to learn, they are not diminishing you. They are handing you something valuable. I know because people told me that early in my career, and I was too young and too certain of myself to fully receive it. I had to learn most of it the hard way anyway. You do not have to.

The five things that work for me are these–real coping mechanisms that you will actually use: A personal board of directors who will tell you the truth. An identity that is bigger than your job title. Professional help when you need it, and you will need it at some point. Healthy coping mechanisms you will actually use, the kind that give the stress somewhere to go. And time away from this work that genuinely turns it off.

None of these are complicated. All of them require intention. The job will not remind you to do them. The job will pull in the opposite direction every chance it gets. That is why you decide now, before the weight accumulates, that you are going to be the kind of provider who is still here twenty years from now with their health reasonably intact and something left in the cup.

Now one question remains, and it is the hardest one in this book. With everything you've just read in mind, let's face it honestly.

Chapter 15: Is This Still Right For You?

I want to start this chapter by telling you something I rarely say out loud.

I believe I was called to this profession. Not in a metaphorical sense. I was raised Catholic, went to Catholic schools from pre-K through college, and at some point during my more devout years I was at an adoration of the Eucharist. People around me were praying, some speaking in tongues, which I never understood. I was sitting quietly. And something came over me. Not a voice exactly. A pull. *Join the rescue squad.* So I did. And here we are.

I do not share that story often. I am sharing it here because this chapter is about the hardest question in this book, which is how you know when it is time to stay and when it is time to go. And for me, the answer lives in that moment. When everything else has told me to leave, something underneath it all has kept pulling me back.

Let me tell you how many times I almost did not come back.

When my father was sick, I was running on empty in every direction at once. Nursing school full time during the day. Volunteering one night a week. Working four nights a week at paid EMS.

Planning a wedding. I had also been elected President and CEO of my volunteer agency, a role I was far too young for (but that is a story for another time). The point is that I was gone. I was always somewhere else. My father worked hard his whole life, and I got that from him, but what that meant in practice was that on his weekends I was either sleeping or working. He got sick. He fought for a year. He died on Father's Day in 2013. And I will never get that time back.

I want to be clear that I am not telling you that story as a unique James Mazza tragedy. I am telling you because it is the honest reality of what this career asks of the people around you. It will ask that of you too. Your family will miss you. Your friends will stop inviting you because you are never available. I had a group of friends from my years working at a grocery store before EMS, all of us close, all of us going for half price apps at Applebee's and hanging out on weekends. Once I was in EMS, that stopped. Our schedules never overlapped again. They were out living their lives and I was sleeping between shifts or working overnight. That world closed.

My father's death forced me to step back from nursing school. I could not keep up with everything I was carrying and something had to give. In the end I do not regret it—I genuinely love EMS and I went on to get my master's degree in Emergency Management and Disaster Planning, so education did not die with that goal.

But at the time it felt like another thing the career had taken.

I was also married by then and missing time with my wife and friends for the same reason I had always missed everything. Sleeping or working. I knew I needed out. What I did not understand yet was that I needed out of the specific agency and position I was in, not out of the industry.

So I left. And I spent a few years moving from job to job outside of EMS, trying to find something that fit—only maintaining a few per-diem shifts per month to keep my skills sharp and my options open. At one point my friend, the man who was my supervisor and stood at my wedding, joked that he could not recommend me for a position anywhere because he knew I would be miserable and leave. He was not wrong. I was miserable every time. Not because the jobs were bad, but because they were not this. Not 911 EMS. Not the thing I had been called to do in that quiet room years before. I eventually got laid off from a job as the office manager of a gun range. I got a paid full-time supervisor position at my volunteer agency, which had always run with a mix of paid staff and volunteers. The die was cast. I stopped fighting it.

The hardest thing to learn is the difference between a bad season and a real ending.

I thought I knew the difference. After leading my agency through COVID, I stepped back to part time EMS and took a remote position at a healthcare company. I thought I was fine. I had done the hard thing and come out the other side. Then I started crying watching movies I loved. Not sad movies. Movies I had seen a dozen times. I did not know why it was happening. Eventually I connected with a disaster support hotline worker and we figured it out together. Survivor's guilt. I had led people through something devastating and then walked away while they were still in it. I was not there when it mattered and some part of me could not reconcile that, even though logically I knew I had done what I needed to do.

The field staff told me afterward that even though I was second in command they felt like I was running it. I always deflected that. Still do. But I am writing it down here because it matters to the point I am trying to make, which is this: you cannot always see what a bad season looks like from inside it. Talk to someone. Your board of directors, a therapist, a hotline worker at two in the morning. They can see what you cannot. They helped me figure out it was a season and not an ending. It might be an ending for you. There is no shame in that either.

I have watched people leave this profession and I have learned something different from each of them.

One of our paid staff walked away after a child died on a call. He was a father of two. He had been doing this for years and that call overflowed his cup completely. He was done and he knew it and he honored that knowledge by leaving. That was the right call for him. Others were never in this for the long haul, and that is fine too. EMS is a stepping stone for a lot of people who go on to become doctors, nurses, paramedics, cops, firefighters. Some of the best providers I have ever worked with were using this job as their foundation for something else. I was supposed to be one of them. This was meant to be a stepping stone toward law enforcement.

The profession drives people out. That is the truth of it. There is no meaningful upward mobility, the pay does not reflect the work, and the best and brightest eventually look around and do the math. I have been able to stay because I have a spouse who earns more than I do and has never once made me feel guilty about dedicating my life to a field that will never make us rich. I know how lucky that makes me. Not everyone has that and the profession loses good people because of it.

What has staying cost me? My father's weekends. Friends I stopped being able to keep up with. A sleep schedule I may never fully recover. A body that has been carrying the weight of night shifts and bad meals and accumulated stress for close to two decades. I am still working on all of it.

What has staying given me?

Purpose. A reason to get up that has nothing to do with a paycheck. A way to leave something behind in this world that does not require me to pass on my DNA. This book is part of that. The providers I have trained and mentored and pushed and supported are part of that. The woman who hugged me at the car show is part of that.

I will not be having children. That is a choice I have made and I am at peace with it. What I have instead is a legacy built in the people who came through this profession alongside me or because of me. That is not a consolation prize. That is the whole point.

So here is what I want to leave you with as you close this book.

I did not write this to scare you. I wrote it because you deserved the truth before you walked through the door, not after you had already been through it. The textbooks will teach you medicine. This was supposed to teach you everything else.

If you are still here after reading all of this, something in you wants this. Trust that. It has never steered me wrong even when everything around me was telling me to go a different direction.

And if you want to understand where all of this came from, if you want to understand the history and the soul of the profession you are entering, go read *American Sirens* by Kevin

Hazzard. It is the true story of the first paramedics in America. The first intubation ever performed outside of a hospital was done by a person of color in Pittsburgh in the late 1960s. I did not know that until I read it. I suspect you did not know it either. That history belongs to you now. This profession belongs to you now.

Take care of it.

Dedication

To my parents.

My mother, who took the photos I pretended not to want and kept them anyway. Because of her I have proof of where this all started, a kid in an oversized coat on a front porch who had no idea what was coming.

My father, who never stopped asking about the calls the way a curious stranger would, who built in me the work ethic that this career demands, and who laid the foundation I have been building on ever since. I carry him with me every shift.

To my wife Kristen, who has never once made me feel guilty for choosing a profession that asks everything of the people who love someone in it. And to Apollo, and to Vader, who is no longer here but whose presence I still feel. My dogs have always known when I needed to decompress before I did.

To the seventy dedicated members of Montclair Ambulance Unit, from the newest per-diem EMT to the Board President who pushed me to apply for NJ Task Force 1 Urban Search and Rescue and recommended me when I did. He gave me the chance. It is the honor of my professional life to serve as your leader. Every version of what I have become in this profession happened because of what this organization asked of me and trusted me with.

To Matthew Streger, from whom I shamelessly borrowed the concept of the personal board of directors. He borrowed it from someone else. That is how the best ideas travel.

And to Joey Cofone, my best friend since the first grade, a genuine artist and the person who never stopped pushing me to see this industry and this profession differently. This book exists in part because of those conversations.

To my personal board of directors. You know who you are. You answer when I call, you tell me the truth when I need to hear it, and you have never once let me figure out the hard stuff alone. This career would have broken me without you.

To everyone I have crossed paths with in EMS. Some of you I call friends. Some were coworkers I have not spoken to in years. Some I see once a year at a conference and pick up right where we left off. All of you contributed to this book in ways you will never fully know. Every conversation, every call, every moment of watching someone do this job well or badly taught me something that ended up on these pages.

This one is for all of you.

About the Author

James Mazza, MA, is the Chief of Emergency Medical Services at Montclair Ambulance Unit, an independent nonprofit 911 agency serving Montclair and Cedar Grove, New Jersey. He has spent nearly twenty years in prehospital emergency care, holding progressive leadership roles across multiple agencies before assuming his current position overseeing a team of seventy certified EMTs responding to more than 5,500 calls annually.

James began his EMS career in 2006 as a volunteer with the Nutley Volunteer Emergency and Rescue Squad, where he would eventually serve as Assistant Chief. He simultaneously built a fifteen-year career with Paramus Emergency Medical Services, earning multiple Life-Saving Awards for CPR saves. He holds a Bachelor of Arts in Political Science from Seton Hall University and a Master of Arts in Emergency and Disaster Management from American Public University, where he was inducted into the Epsilon Pi Phi Emergency Management Honor Society.

He is a Deployable Logistics Specialist with NJ Task Force 1, one of twenty-eight FEMA nationally deployable Urban Search and Rescue teams, and has deployed to large-scale disaster operations including Hurricane Helene in North Carolina. He serves as a Staging Officer for the New Jersey EMS Task Force Central Region and sits on the Community Board of Trustees at Mountainside Medical Center.

James was named Prehospital Administrator of the Year by the New Jersey Department of Health Office of Emergency Medical Services in 2024 and EMS Advocate of the Year by the National Association of Emergency Medical Technicians in 2025. He serves as Director at Large for the International Association of EMS Chiefs and as NAEMT State Advocacy Coordinator for New Jersey.

He lives in northern New Jersey with his wife Kristen and their German Shepherd, Apollo.

www.ingramcontent.com/pod-product-compliance
Lightning Source LLC
LaVergne TN
LVHW010737061126
851857LV00014B/1527
* 9 7 9 8 9 9 7 8 1 2 2 0 1 *